I0795250

MY FRIEND WITH HEALTH NEEDS

MY FRIEND WITH ADHD

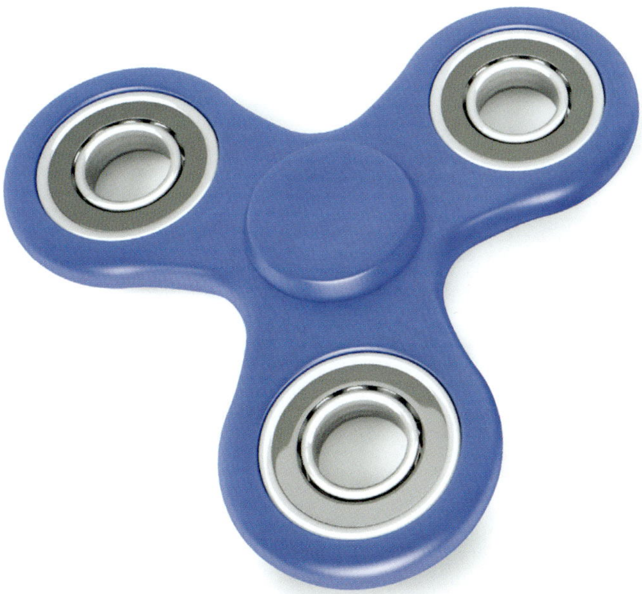

by Elizabeth Andrews

Cody Koala

An Imprint of Pop!
popbooksonline.com

Hello! My name is

Cody Koala

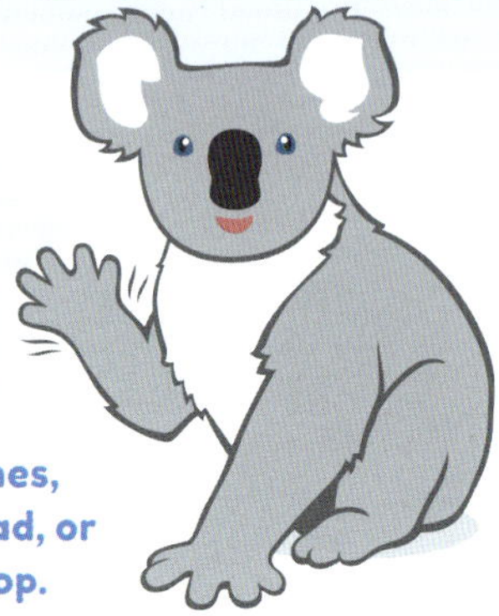

This book is filled with videos, puzzles, games, and more! Scan the QR codes* while you read, or visit the website below to make this book pop.

popbooksonline.com/ADHD

*Scanning QR codes requires a web-enabled smart device with a QR code reader app and a camera.

abdobooks.com

Published by Pop!, a division of ABDO, PO Box 398166, Minneapolis, Minnesota 55439. Copyright ©2024 by Abdo Consulting Group, Inc. International copyrights reserved in all countries. No part of this book may be reproduced in any form without written permission from the publisher. Cody Koala™ is a trademark and logo of Pop!.

Printed in the United States of America, North Mankato, Minnesota.

102023
012024

THIS BOOK CONTAINS RECYCLED MATERIALS

Cover Photo: Shutterstock Images
Interior Photos: Shutterstock Images; Getty Images
Editor: Grace Hansen
Series Designer: Victoria Bates

Library of Congress Control Number: 2023938796

Publisher's Cataloging-in-Publication Data

Names: Andrews, Elizabeth, author.
Title: My friend with ADHD / by Elizabeth Andrews
Description: Minneapolis, Minnesota : Pop!, 2024 | Series: My friend with health needs | Includes online resources and index
Identifiers: ISBN 9781098245276 (lib. bdg.) | ISBN 9781098245832 (ebook)
Subjects: LCSH: Friendship--Juvenile literature. | Attention-deficit hyperactivity disorder--Juvenile literature. | Attention-deficit-disordered youth--Juvenile literature. | Social acceptance--Juvenile literature.
Classification: DDC 618.928589--dc23

Table of Contents

Chapter 1

Overwhelmed

Maya's mom told her to clean her room. But Maya doesn't know where to start. There are clothes pouring out of the closet, books on the bed, and toys on the floor. Maya gets **overwhelmed** and cries.

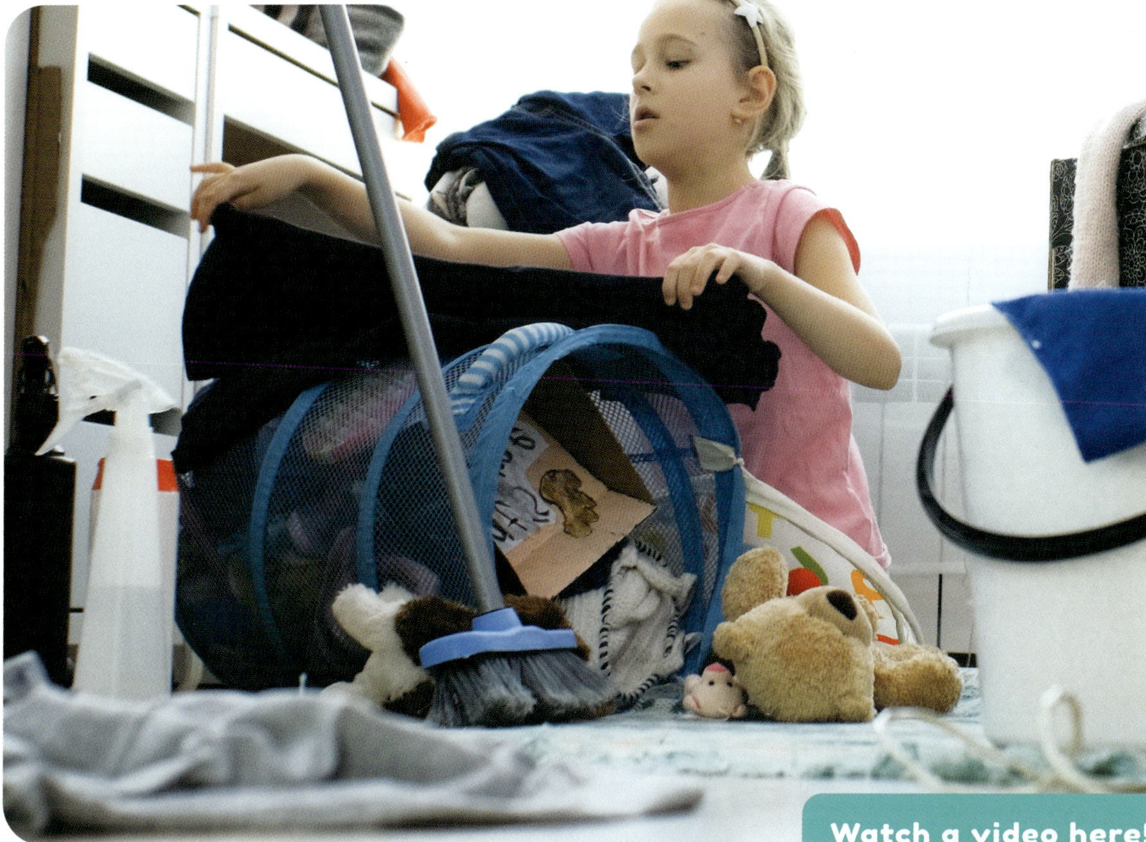

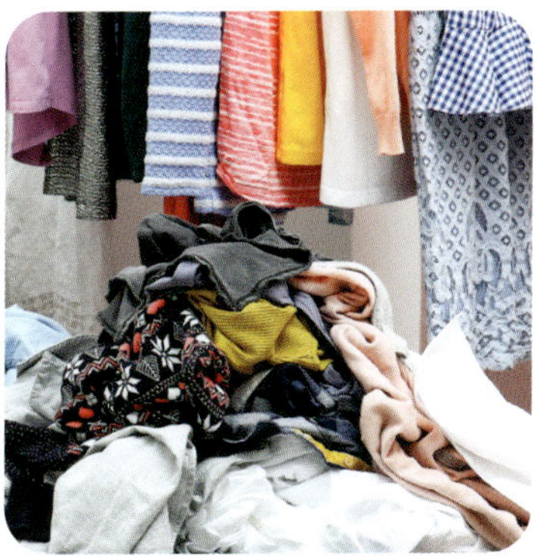

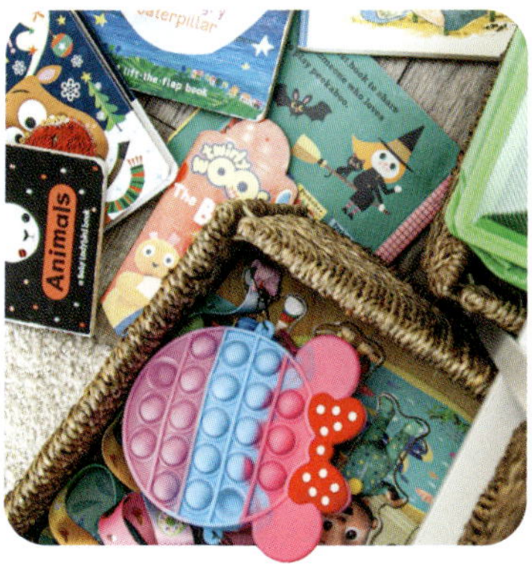

Watch a video here!

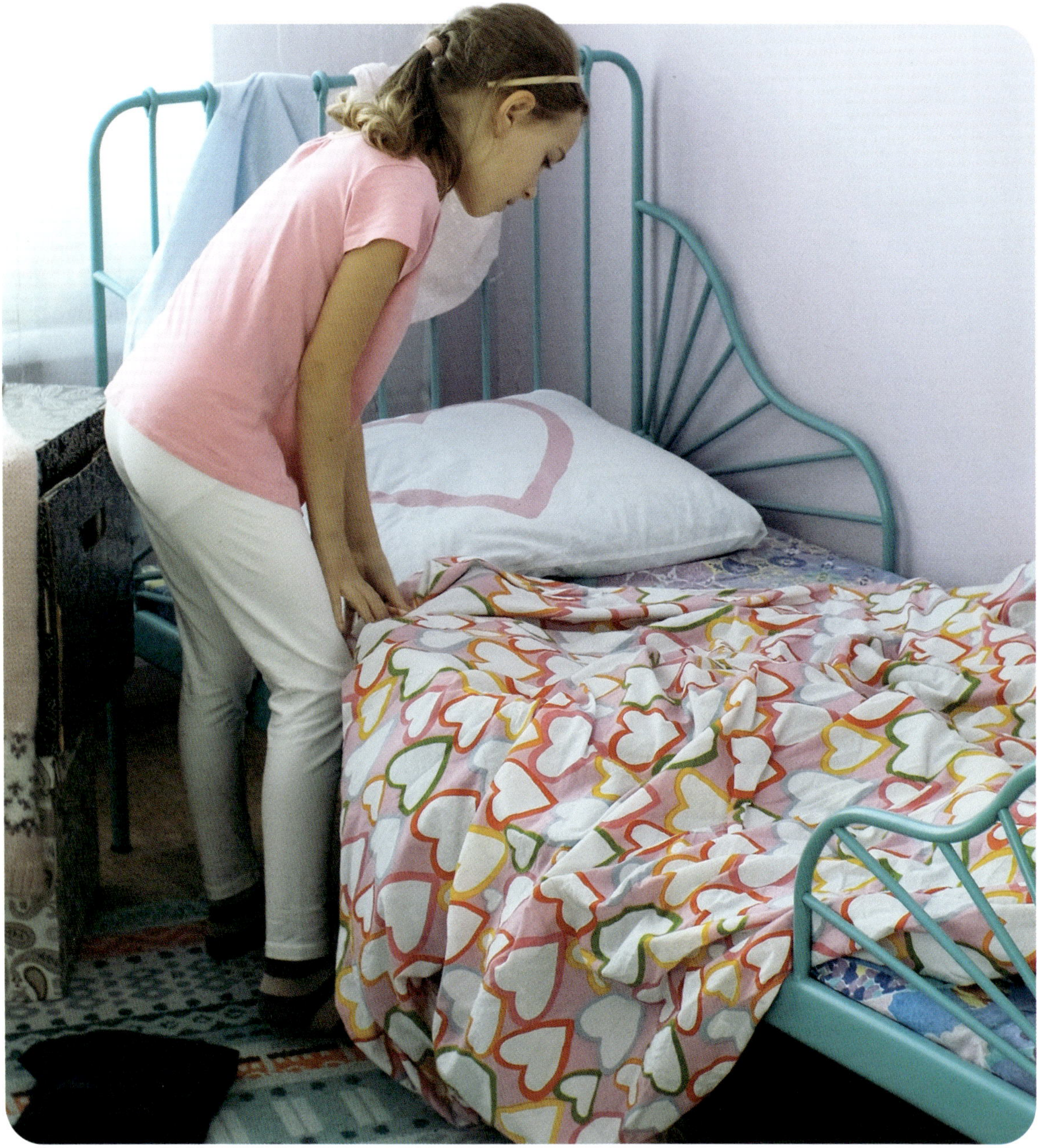

Maya knows her ADHD makes starting a big project hard. Maya's mom helps her break down the cleaning into small, easy steps. Maya's room is clean in time for a pizza dinner!

Chapter 2

What Is ADHD?

ADHD stands for attention-deficit/hyperactivity **disorder**. It is a disorder that can make it hard for a person to listen, **focus**, and control their behaviors.

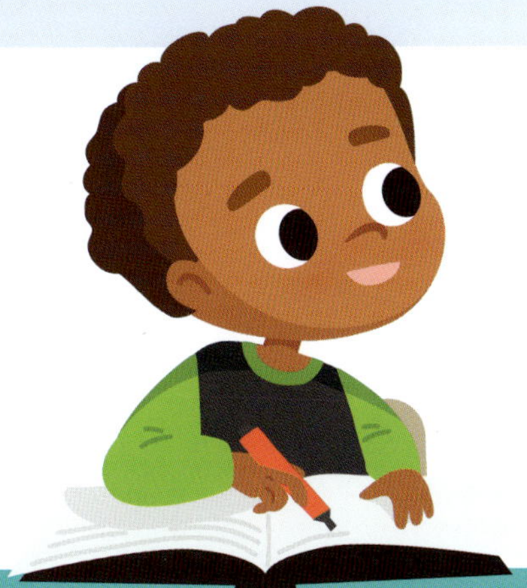

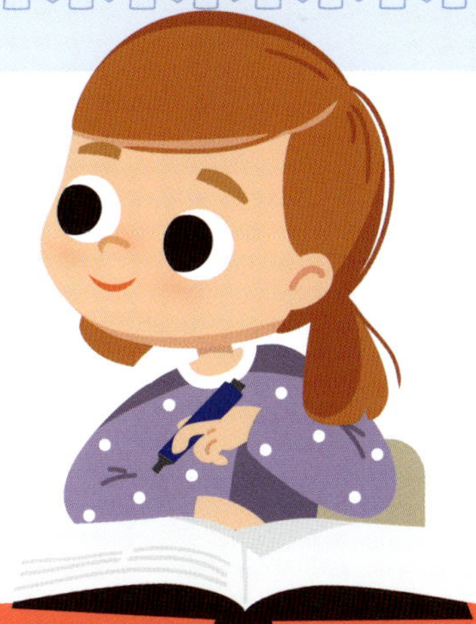

ADHD in BOYS

- Acting without thinking
- Very active
- Trouble paying attention
- Forceful with body
- Disruptive

ADHD in GIRLS

- Shy or not social
- Nervous or fearful
- Trouble paying attention
- Forceful with body
- Impatient

It is sometimes easier to spot ADHD in boys than girls. It's more noticeable when boys interrupt or can't sit still. To find ADHD in girls, teachers and parents have to be knowledgeable about the disorder.

Learn more here!

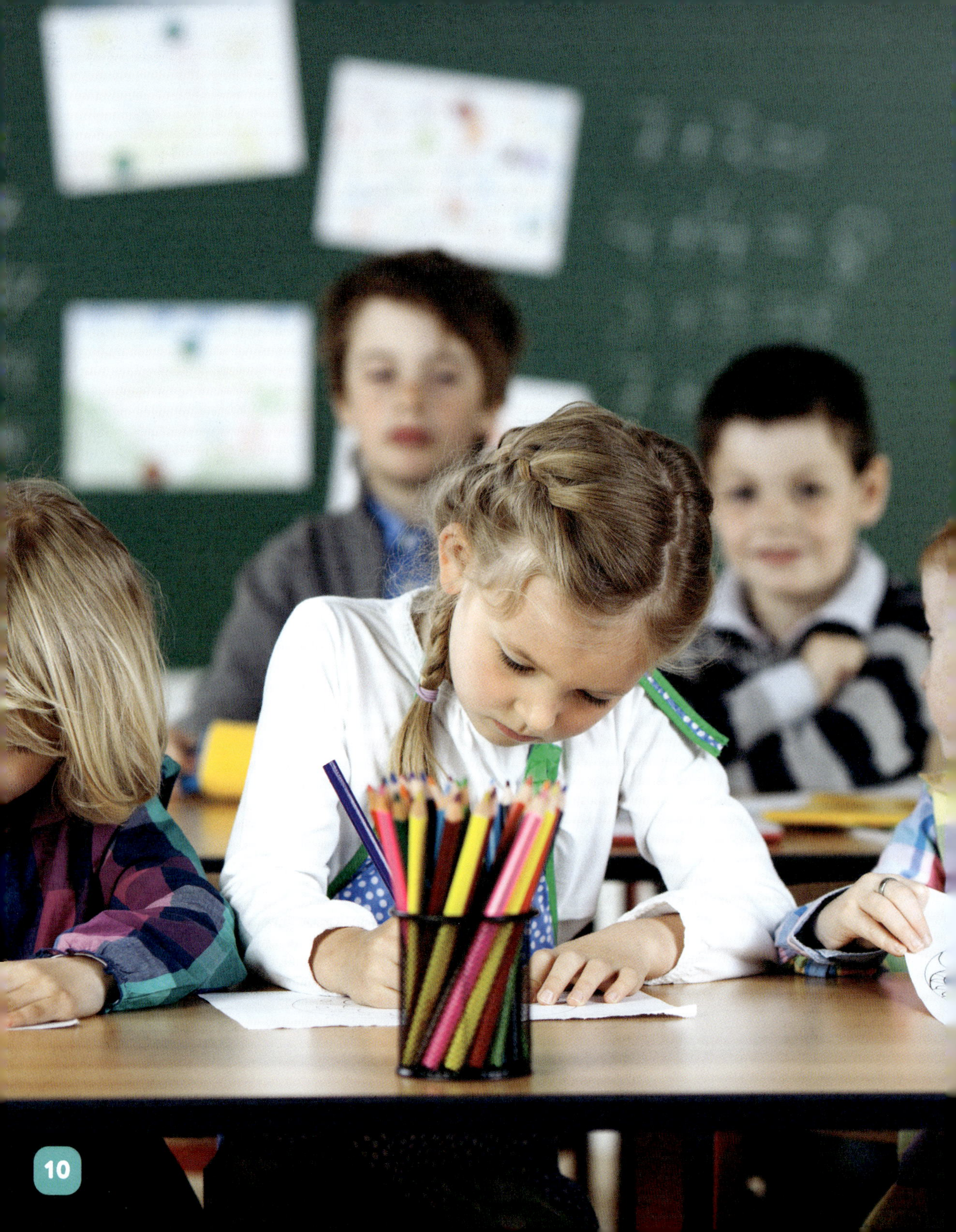

Any student can have trouble paying attention in class. But kids with ADHD struggle with it every day. They have to work harder to stay focused on a task and get it done.

It's easy for kids with ADHD to get distracted by a bird outside a classroom window or noise in the hallway.

Chapter 3

Types of ADHD

There are two types of ADHD. The **inattentive** type causes a person to have trouble **focusing** and staying organized. A person with this type might lose things or struggle to follow directions.

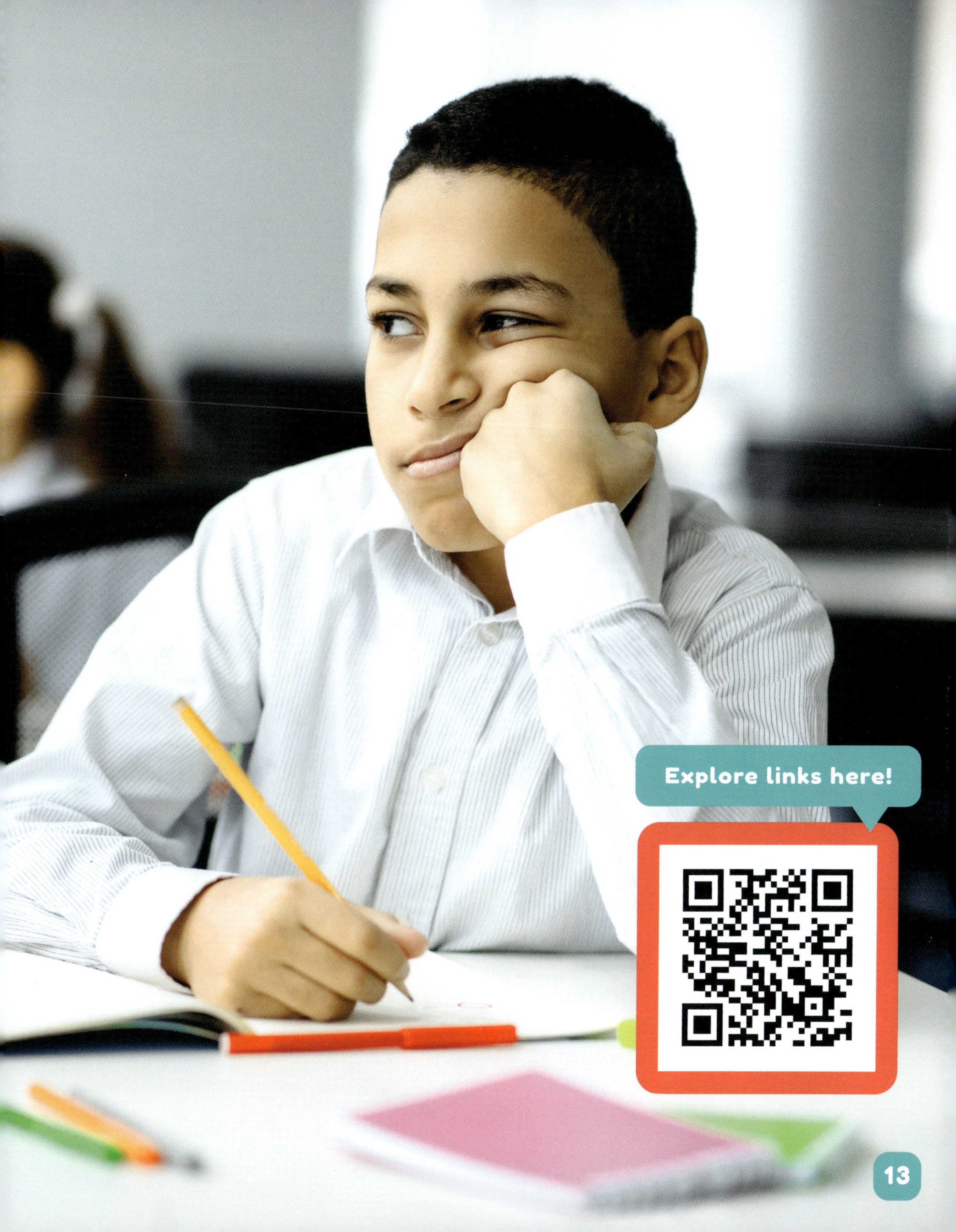

Explore links here!

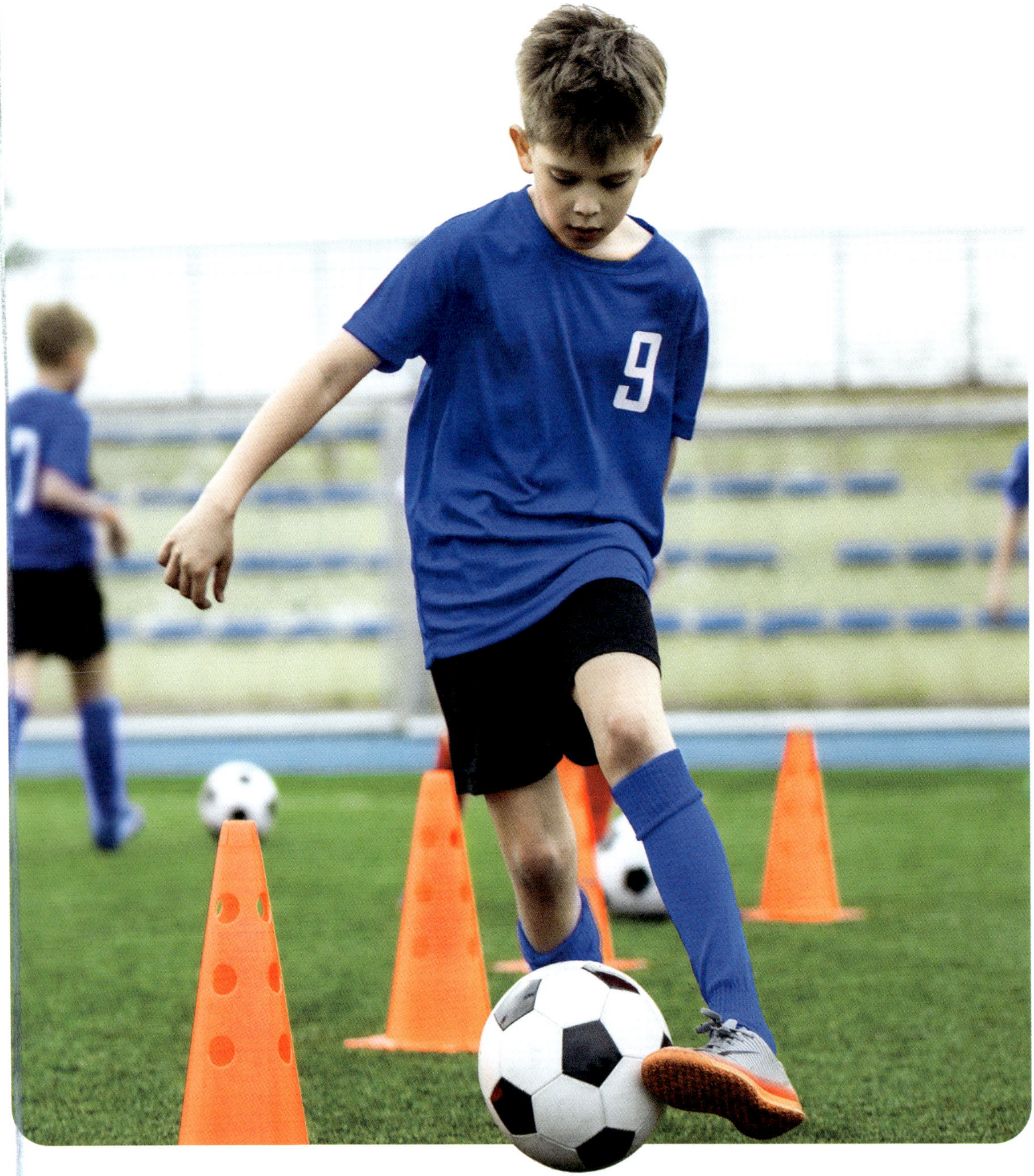
9
7

The hyperactive-**impulsive** type can make it hard for a person to sit still. A person with this type might do or say things without thinking. They might talk a lot or interrupt their teachers and friends.

Chapter 4

ADHD in School

Kids with ADHD can find it hard to sit still during lessons. When a student with ADHD gets in trouble for something they can't control, they can feel **misunderstood**.

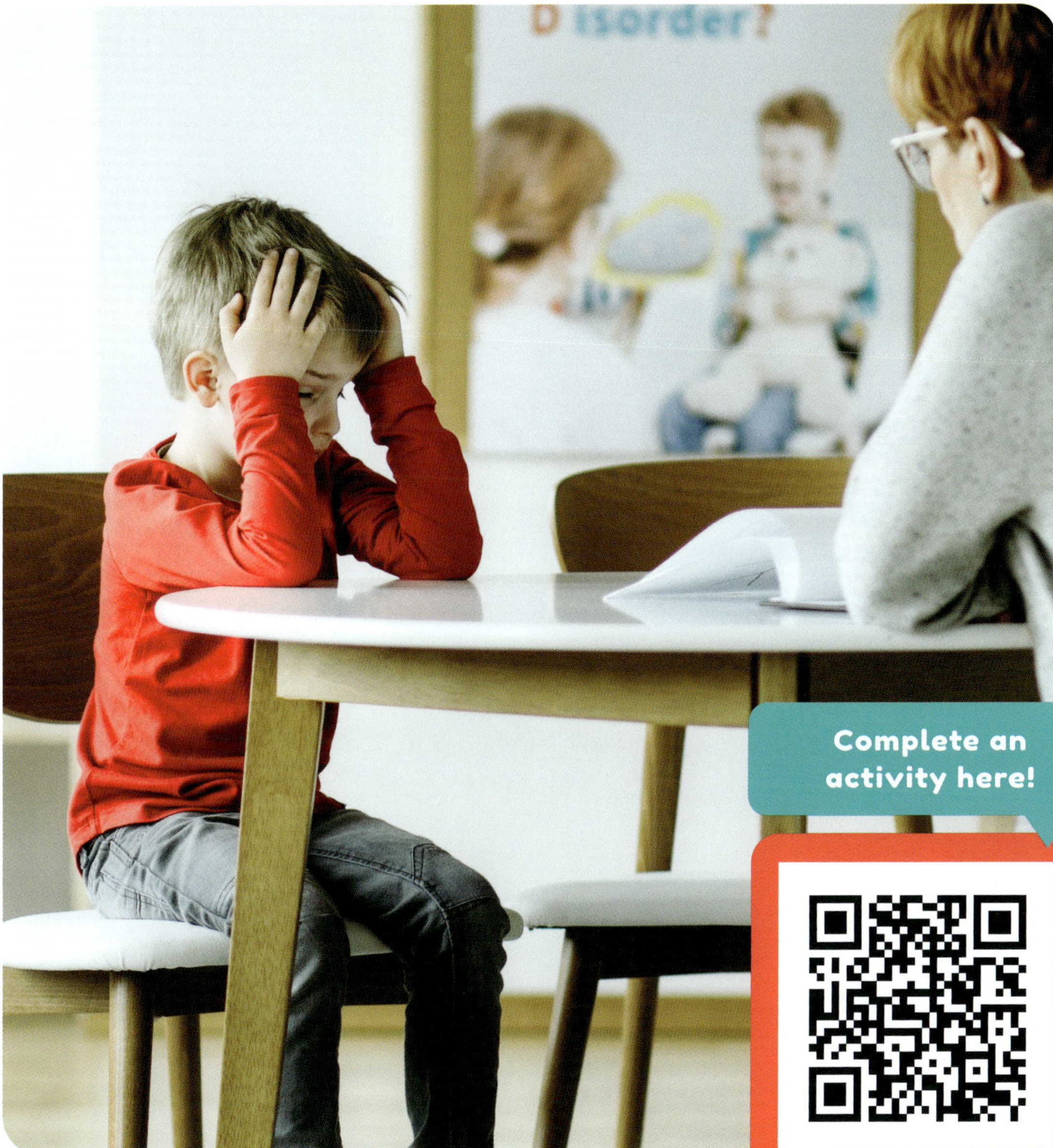

Complete an activity here!

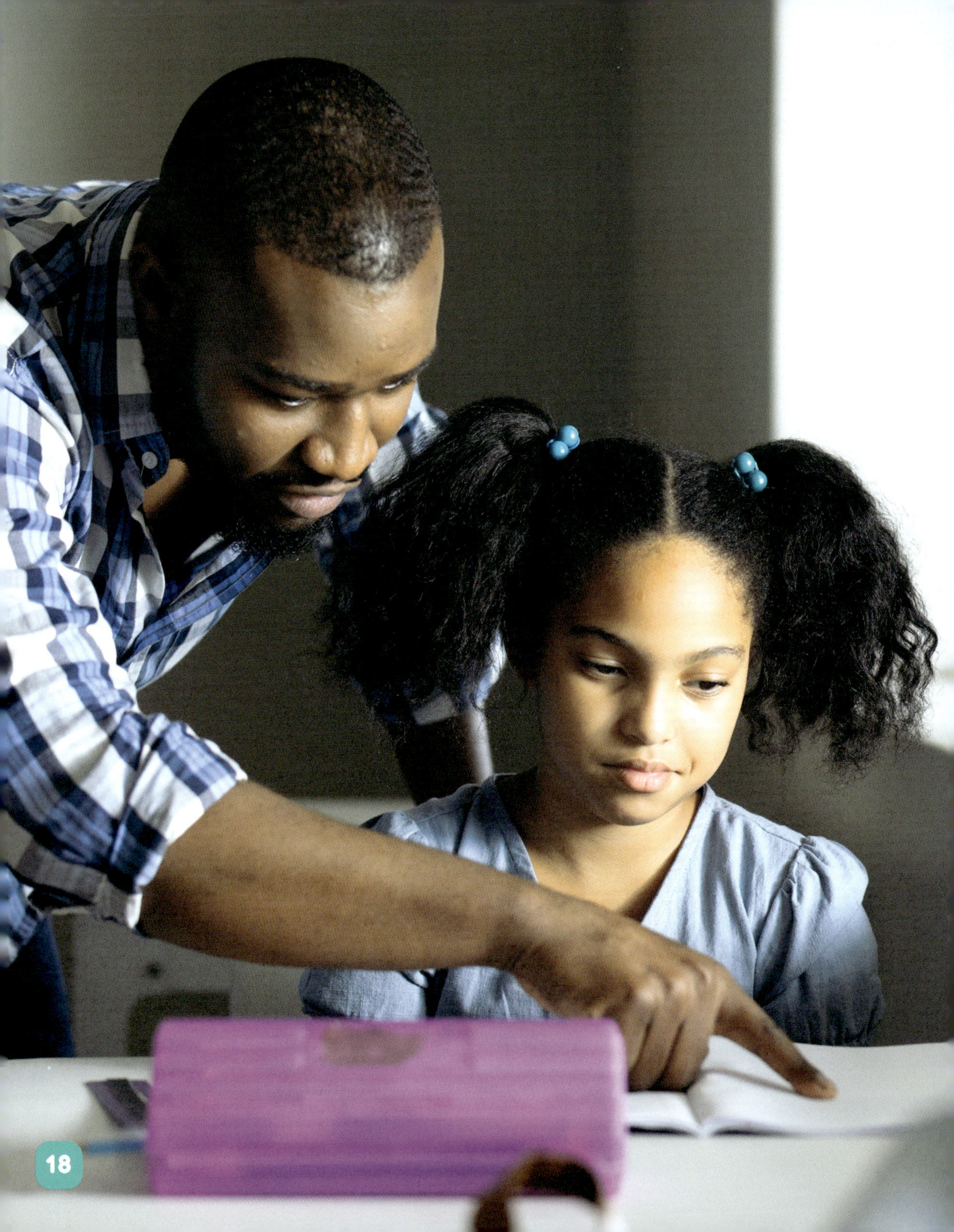

Students with ADHD know that they're supposed to sit quietly in class. But it's more difficult for them. Teachers work with these students to plan ways that help each day run smoothly.

Shortening assignments and taking breaks helps students with ADHD learn better.

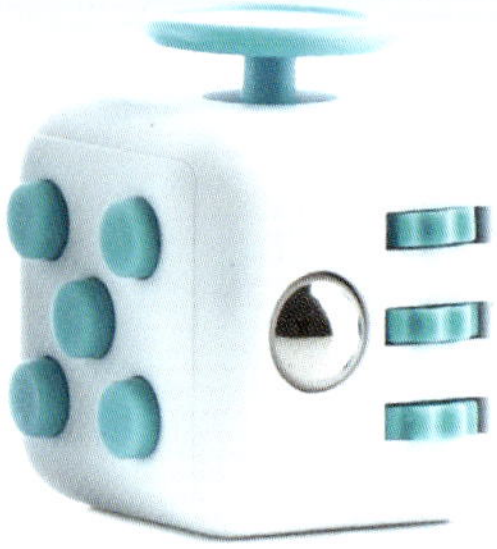

Millions of people have ADHD. Every person **manages** it differently. Some people take medicine to help. Others might use small toys to quietly **focus** their energy. People with ADHD can lead normal, happy lives!

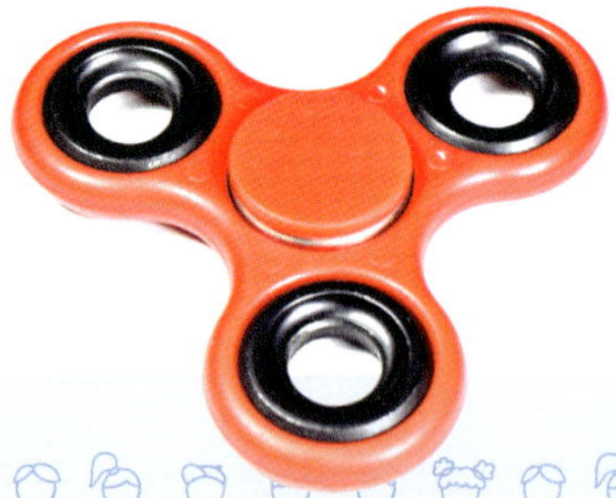

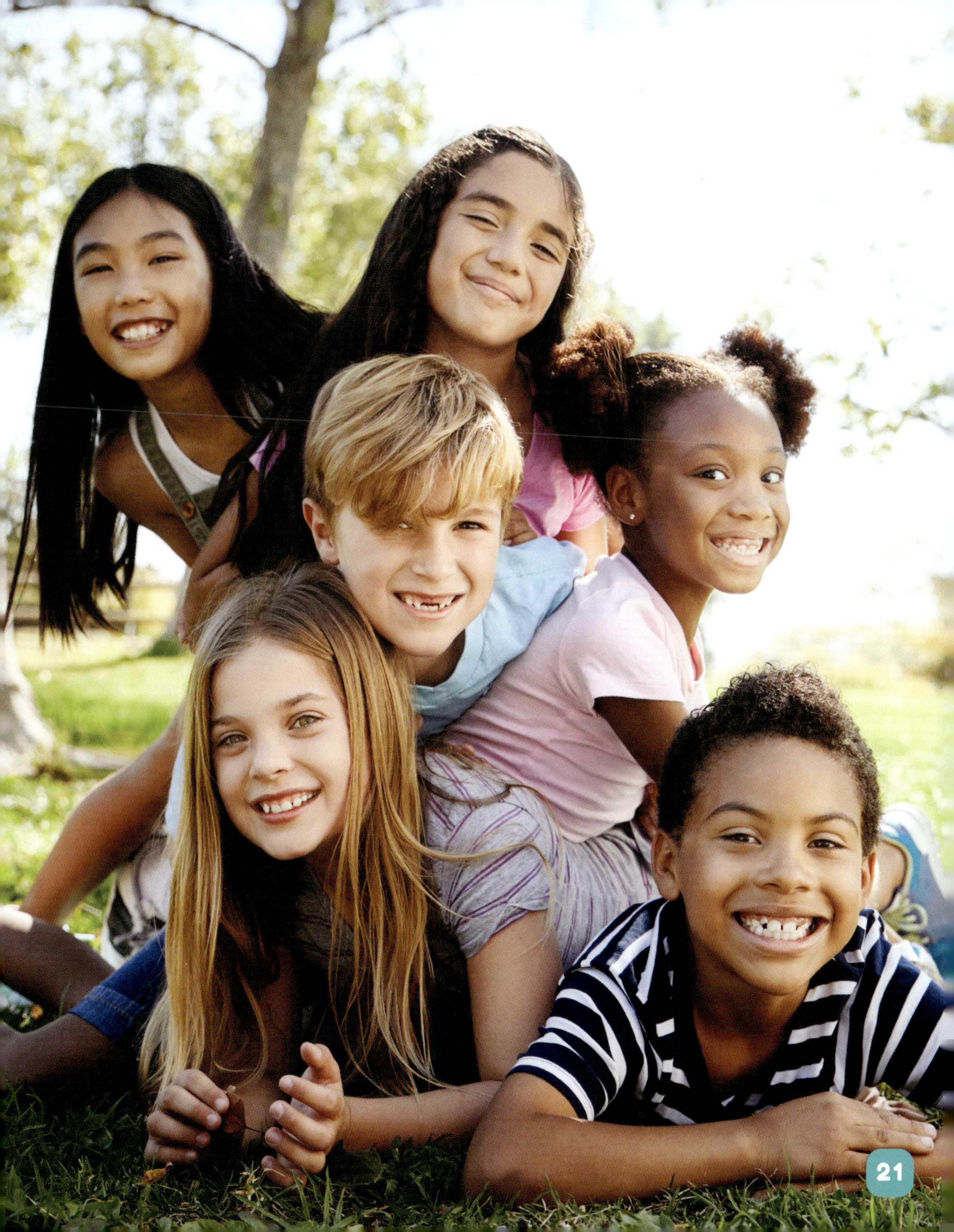

Making Connections

Text-to-Self

Do you or any of your friends have ADHD? If so, how does it make you or them feel?

Text-to-Text

Have you read any other books about a health need that makes school a little more difficult? How is that health need similar to or different from ADHD?

Text-to-World

Come up with three ways schools could improve to help students with ADHD learn better.

Glossary

disorder – a physical or mental sickness or condition.

focus – to give attention or efforts to one thing.

impulsive – acting without thinking or planning.

inattentive – not giving proper attention.

manage – to look after or make decisions about.

misunderstood – not understood correctly.

overwhelmed – to have too much to deal with.

Index

Online Resources

popbooksonline.com

Thanks for reading this Cody Koala book!

This book is filled with videos, puzzles, games, and more! Scan the QR codes* while you read, or visit the website below to make this book pop.

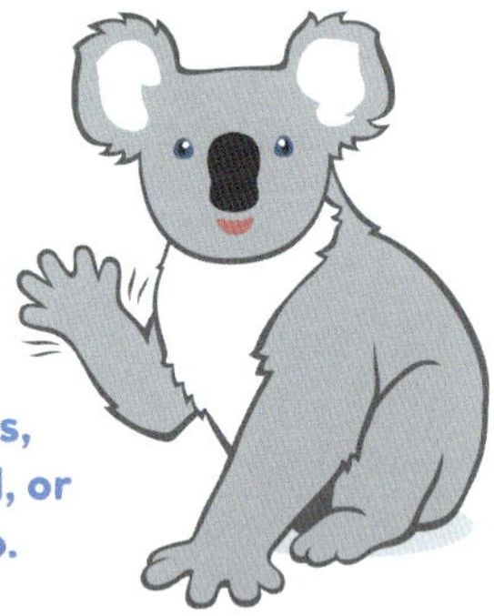

popbooksonline.com/ADHD

*Scanning QR codes requires a web-enabled smart device with a QR code reader app and a camera.